The Binge Fix;

The 7 Techniques To Combat Emotional Eating

By

Patricia J. Myers

Copyright

Table of contents

Introduction

We are, as a whole, to blame for "eating our sentiments" once in a while. At the point when feelings run high, going to nourishment for comfort...well, it works out. To us all.

That is because eating is an intrinsically fulfilling conduct. It should be! We depend on food to make due all things considered. Looking for ways of adapting to pressure is regular, as well, incidentally.

Notwithstanding, we additionally all know that this inclination to adapt through pressure eating, profound eating, anything we desire to call it, isn't precisely solid — truly or intellectually.

One of the issues with emotional eating is that it influences how you feel actually. Indulging can decrease your energy level, cause migraines, and just, for the most part, accompany some distress," says Kasey Kilpatrick, dietitian at Houston Methodist. "That's what the other concerns are, the amount to which settling is difficult, eating doesn't work."

And keeping in mind that there are a lot of eating-related tips and deceives out there to assist with combatting profound eating, Kilpatrick says there's an explanation that these prohibitive food rules don't work for everybody. She likewise prescribes a more useful way to deal with tending to profound eating, and her technique has barely anything to do with food.

"Indeed, even after learning and committing these food rules to memory, for example, restricting ourselves to two snacks each day or not eating past 7 p.m., a significant number of us end up battling with profound eating," says Kilpatrick. "We wish to firstly eradicate this behavior in order to determine the disgrace around it — and afterward we want to utilize a more useful method for tending to it."

Chapter 1

Ditch The Diet

What Is Diet Culture?

Diet culture includes the standards and guidelines that society institutes around our bodies and the food that is suitable to eat. Diet culture most frequently lauds adjusting one's body weight, shape, and measure to decrease.

Diet culture belief is the foundation of slight honor: The unmerited honor that exists in our general public for individuals that were brought into the world with meager bodies.

Key givers of diet culture include:

- Food rules
- A worth on lean, conditioned bodies
- Practice changing the body shape
- Cultural qualities that maintain diet culture include:
- Hairsplitting
- Independence

- Male centric society
- Intensity
- Realism
- Healthism

Diet culture masks itself inside profoundly esteemed standards like really buckling down, regarding the body, and sharing thoughts of prosperity. This makes it extremely challenging to split away from.

Reject The Eating Regimen Mindset

At the point when you find the voice in your mind saying "I should be more slender," or "I just eat clean" Reject the eating regimen attitude by rather posing yourself with these inquiries:

What is the worth of slenderness?

Do my formal food decisions help or harm my general health?

Who stands to gain if I alter my body's size, shape or weight?

Who am I accomplishing slimness for?

What amount of my day am I spending centered around food or my body?

Will being more slender work on the nature of my life? In which ways?

Is there something I could do that could be more significant to my life than the quest for slimness (for

instance, excelling in my vocation or playing with my children)?
Other extraordinary moves toward dismissing the eating routine mindset include:

- Dumping food rules.
- Dispensing with body checking of yourself as well as other people.
- Quit counting calories.

Dumping Food Rules: Food rules are any practices or convictions that there is a correct method for eating. They might be decisions that are pushed by a particular eating regimen. On the other hand, they might be decisions that are far-reaching, for example, eating everything on your plate or what is fitting to eat at specific eating times.

A guideline of Blissful Eating is to jettison food names and diet rules. They accomplish other things to propagate apparent desires, the allurement for taboo food varieties, binging and eating to defy the food rules than advance taking care of oneself and adjusted eating.

The following are 3 Idiot proof Moves toward disposing of Food Rules

1. Make a rundown of your food rules

Presently before you say "I have no food rules… " I believe you should truly assess your considerations and sentiments around food.

Do you allow yourself to eat ANYTHING whenever? If not, you likely have food managers Some place!

Simply monitoring the food rules you have can be a stage towards Testing those food rules to dispose of food rules.

You genuinely must make a rundown of your food rules WITHOUT passing judgment on yourself.

Notice the guidelines you might have as you show them out, yet abstain from scolding yourself for holding any principles.

Here are some normal food rules I see from clients:

- No eating after 7 pm.
- No pastries during the week.
- The carbs are awful. Keep away from it at all costs.
- 1 dull carb each day.
- Just 1 organic product each day is permitted.

- Drink lemon water or apple juice vinegar each day.
- Pick the bread container or liquor while eating out.
- No additional sugar in any food sources.
- Just eat 0% yogurt.

Your food rules can be any convictions, contemplations, or sentiments you have about food. Periodically food rules are affected by past weight control plans that you've attempted. You may not remember it as a food rule since it's become so ingrained in the manner you eat.

Attempt to be straightforward with yourself as you make a rundown of food rules you clutch. You can continuously add more food rules as they jump into your head over the long run.

2. Request your food rules from least demanding to hardest to break

Since you have a rundown of food controls now is the ideal time to begin breaking them. The subsequent stage can be a challenge. From my involvement with working with clients, I view it as least demanding to manage your food rules with a precise methodology. Rather than me saying "presently go eat anything you desire," it's more straightforward to challenge your food leads each in turn.

How we do that is to structure your food rules from your thought process which will be simplest to break to the most troublesome.

It very well may be overpowering to disrupt your food guidelines, so beginning with the most straightforward can make the interaction somewhat less difficult for you.

How do you have any idea what food rules are the least demanding for you to break?

It's an individual decision and it truly relies upon what convictions you hold most grounded.

Suppose three of your food rules are…

- Eat just 1 bland carb each day
- Stay away from all additional sugar
- Eat just 1 serving of organic produce each day

It might be hard for you to add more added sugar into your eating routine assuming you've believed that additional sugar is genuinely horrendous for your health for a long time. All things being equal, it might be simpler for you to defy the norm "Eat just 1 serving of organic product each day" since the natural product contains different supplements and regular sugar.

3. Challenge Your Food Rules

Presently the tomfoolery starts… we will challenge your food controls individually to dispose of food rules. This is likewise a stage that requires a ton of personalization.

How we're going to fundamentally challenge your food rules is to scrutinize their legitimacy and work on rethinking your contemplations.

Individually, for each food rule you have, ask yourself:

- Is there any logical proof to help your food run the show?
- Does this food government sound sensible and additionally maintainable?
- Could you at any point legitimately pick apart this food rule?

However, then, at that point, challenge your thinking and supplant it with a more consistent

- We should accept an illustration of the food rule: "Eat just 1 bland carb each day."
- Pssst - here's an introduction to carbs!

Ask yourself:

- Is there any logical proof to help by just eating 1 dull sugar each day?
- Is eating just 1 boring carb each day reasonable as well as feasible?
- Does it seem OK for my body to eat just 1 boring sugar each day?
- You may likewise wish to truly challenge your food rule right now. For this situation, have a go at eating more than 1 serving of boring carbs each day and perceive how you feel.

This is the very thing you might find when you pose yourself these inquiries to reexamine your food rule with a more coherent idea…

There is no logical proof that recommends I ought to just eat 1 serving of boring carbs each day. My mind expects no less than 150 grams of carbs each day to ideally work.

I frequently want carbs before dinnertime assuming that I just eat one bland carb each day, so it's not exceptionally practical for me, nor maintainable.

The point is when I eat more than 1 dull carb each day I have more energy, fewer desires, and fewer binges, so it doesn't check out for me to restrict myself like this.

Given your impressions of what works for your body and from logical proof that you might explore or ask an expert, you can consistently see that you've disproven your food rule.

If you haven't yet genuinely attempted to challenge your food rule, right now is an ideal opportunity. How would you feel when you eat more than 1 boring carb each day?

Rehearsing food impartiality: Food lack of bias is the comprehension that no single food holds better dietary or virtue over another.

This thought frequently gets pushback in a universe of diet culture, a framework that advocates for food varieties that change the body weight, shape, or size.

- It is accomplished through practicing food lack of bias:
- recognizing and excusing food rules
- fostering a relationship of trust with our bodies.
- excusing rules about balance.
- distinguishing and presenting ourselves to fear food varieties to diminish nervousness around unambiguous food varieties.

- buying, preparing and partaking in a wide range of food varieties.

Disposing of body checking of yourself as well as other people Not many individuals overcome a day without searching in a mirror, surveying the attack of their garment, or considering their general appearance.

Body checking, in the period of constantly refreshed selfies, might be more normal now than at any time in recent memory. Be that as it may, how can you say whether it's sound — or on the other hand assuming that it's turned into an enthusiastic way of behaving?

What is body checking?

Body checking is the propensity for looking for data about your body's weight, shape, size, or appearance.

In the same way as other ways of behaving, the body taking a look exists on a continuum. It can go from totally abstaining from taking a gander at your body to relaxed checking as a component of your arrangements for the afternoon, to habitual and restless check-and-check-again conduct circles.

What's viewed as impulsive?

Everybody looks at the mirror in the workplace bathroom before a gathering or in their restroom before a Zoom home base to make certain there's no spinach in their teeth. Bunches of individuals step on a scale like clockwork to ensure they're in a sound weight territory for them. Furthermore, a lot of individuals take estimations or when selfies to follow their wellness processes.

As indicated by research, however, this can prompt gloomy sentiments when done time and again. Impulsively squeezing free skin, estimating body parts, gauging yourself on numerous occasions every day, and other observing ways of behaving can all wind up demolishing your temperament.

Body checking can become risky if it:

- slows down your capacity to think obviously or concentrate
- takes up a lot of your time
- makes you stop or stringent limit your eating
- makes issues in your work, scholarly, or individual life
- makes you seclude yourself from others
- turns into a method for controlling trepidation and uneasiness about your body

- Body checking is normal among individuals, everything being equal. However, a 2019 study by trusted Sources discovered that for individuals who recognize themselves as ladies, body checking is probably going to cause body disappointment, regardless of which portion of the body is being observed.

Furthermore, a 2018 meta-analysis recommends that urgent body checking can leave you feeling more disappointed with your body and may deteriorate your temperament.
It might likewise prompt a wrong or ridiculous perspective on your weight and body shape.
Instructions to lessen the body taking a look at ways of behaving
Assuming body checking is adding to your concerns or obstructing your everyday life, you might need to think about a portion of these systems to decrease your reliance on this way of dealing with hardship or stress:

- Have some time off from web-based entertainment. In a recent report, scientists found that posting selfies and other web-based entertainment ways of behaving can deteriorate nerves about body size and shape.

- Notice what compels you to need to body check. Sorting out what circumstances incite the drive can assist you with keeping away from those triggers or tracking down ways of decreasing their effect.
- Monitor the taking a look at ways of behaving for a day. Taking note of how frequently your body checks in a 24-hour term might assist you with understanding how long you spend on the way of behaving. It can likewise assist you with setting an objective for diminishing the times you're making it happen.
- Take a stab at a novel, a new thing to oversee uneasiness. When you know when you're powerless against body checking, you can set up some elective survival methods to attempt all things considered.
- Think about chatting with a specialist. If body checking is expanding your tension, bringing down your confidence, or obstructing your everyday life, it's really smart to chat with an expert specialist — whether it's on the web, face to face, or in a

social scene. A prepared specialist might have the option to assist you with grasping your inspirations and foster better methodologies for dealing with your concerns.

- Quit counting calories On the off chance that you dread putting on weight, console yourself by showing up just one time each week. Ensure you tip the scales simultaneously consistently, ideally in the first part of the day after you go to the restroom. It tends to be a major help to see that you are not putting on weight as you go through this interaction.

Stage 1: Practice possibly eating when hungry

Get to know what to crave and what that feels like for you in your body. Comprehending that yearning Is a typical sensation like utilizing the bathroom or feeling drowsy by the end of the day's end. It's anything but an indication of anything being incorrect or that you need to snap right into it right away, it's a sign that your body is prepared for food at some point. Working on feeling hungry for a 30-an hours before eating each time will assist you with flattening dread or uneasiness in regards to the craving, and see that it is your partner in controlling food consumption, not a "terrible" vibe that should be kept away from and forestalled.

Stage 2: Intend to eat 3-4 dinners per day

Assuming you eat little feasts and snacks over the day, help your admission at dinners with the goal that you can get more hours between dinners easily. Adding more food to lunch can quit thinking about nourishment for the day and assist you with discarding a midday nibble.

As of now, it's no issue by any stretch of the imagination if you continue gauging, estimating, and logging all that you eat for consolation.

Stage 3: Quit gauging/counting foods grown from the ground

Assuming you've been steadily following, you are most likely mindful that new vegetables and natural products don't contribute huge amounts of calories to your feasts. Assuming you feel prepared, let go of logging the calories in your leafy foods. This will imply that the calorie complete you see is somewhat not as much as the thing you are eating, however, you won't utilize a specific number to eat up to any longer, you will utilize your hunger prompts, so it's

OK on the off chance that that number is somewhat off. Having a rough estimate can assist with holding you back from getting excessively far out of your usual range of familiarity.

Stage 4: Lose the log after every feast

You can continue estimating or following different food varieties, simply keep no long-lasting record. Dispose of your information toward the day's end. It frequently isn't helping you in any capacity to have a long time of food information recorded. What is important is at this very moment.

I suggest setting a base protein and fat admission to hold back nothing feast, which assists with consuming adjusted dinners and remaining fulfilled. For the vast majority, getting no less than 30 grams of protein and 15 grams of fat for every dinner is a decent spot to begin for 3-4 feasts per day, however for a great many people that will be the base. Then, add other nutritious food sources you appreciate to balance the feast and feel fulfilled. Heap on the broccoli, crunch an apple and have some quinoa assuming that is what you like.

In particular, don't become involved with keeping track of who's winning and attempting to eat less because of the more unhealthy supper you had the previous evening. Simply start at the following dinner with a fresh start, arriving at those essentials and adding different food sources to arrive at fulfillment. This assists your psyche with remaining fixed on the current second and gives the culpability-throwing diet mindset a quick kick in the butt.

Stage 5: Work on eyeballing food-explicitly protein!

You're presumably acclimated with what food sources and divides you're most frequently eating to arrive at your objective protein numbers. As of now, you can eyeball the number of ounces of meat on your plate with sensible exactness. If you feel prepared, let yourself gauge bits to hit your protein focus without utilizing the scale to weigh it like clockwork. A few things will normally be divided for you at any rate like eggs, for instance, or individual Greek yogurts.

To emphasize, if you're involving yearning and satiety as your essential aide, whether you have 4 ounces or 5 ounces of chicken bosom at lunch today, it won't make any difference over the long haul because your body will change hunger and fulfillment to your changing energy admission and requirements. For the vast majority, a "palm" of meat turns out great.

Stage 6: Get adaptable

You could have previously quit utilizing the following programming yet On the off chance that not, inquire as to whether it's truly doing anything for you. You're utilizing rationale to ensure you're in the ideal ballpark for protein to remain fulfilled, and you're eating entire food sources over the day. You're allowing appetite to sign you that it's a chance to eat

I urge you to allow yourself to have adaptability, feast by dinner and step by step, even week to week. Adaptable eating works better than an unbending nature. Take into account the ups and downs that will adjust. On the off chance that you have an extraordinary occasion or need dessert, take a gander at it to the general extent of your eating routine - uncommon special cases in energy consumption don't make an individual addition or shed pounds assuming that your propensities are sound more often than not. Eat just when you've been eager for a 30-an hour, pick practically all entire, high supplement thick food sources, and stick to 3-4 feasts each day with everyone having a few proteins and fat remembered for them.

As you travel through this interaction, recollect to not overreact at little fluctuations on the scale, as the normal individual differs every day inside a scope of around 4 pounds. Be that as it may, on the off chance that the pattern is going up throughout 3 a month, rather than dashing back to counting calories, consider dialing down the calorie thickness of your feasts by diminishing segments of fats and picking more vegetables and organic products rather than grain items or starches like potatoes. Likewise, do a twofold verify whether you can lessen fluid calories, sugars, or handled food varieties.

Diet Versus Way of life Change

We've all heard it. "It's anything but an eating regimen. It represents a shift in way of life,but does it really entail?

Attributes of diets include:

- Rules and limitations about food
- Interest in an expansion in workout
- A commitment to better "well-being"
- A change in the body as well as the brain
- Vows to decrease body size

- Way of life changes is frequently connected with commitments of:

Precisely the same standards and guidelines as diets. But the way of life changes guarantees to be economical until the end of your life.

Way of life changes, very much like eating regimens are regularly not practical. This is a misleading story intended to persuade us that if we "simply turn out more enthusiastically for a more extended timeframe" at our prohibitive conduct we will succeed.

Can we just look at things objectively? Way of life change turned into the popular new term for eating less when the whole world understood that diets don't work.

However even though individuals understood that diets didn't create the practical weight reduction diet culture guaranteed them for a long time, we became frantic for one more road to slimness, and the honor it gave.

A great many people will have weight reduction bounce back in the span of an extended time of finishing their eating regimen.

Next time somebody discusses "way of life transforms" I believe you should ask yourself: "Does it have rules?" Provided that this is true it is an eating regimen. I need to clarify that conditions like "with some restraint" are additionally administered, and are additionally essential for diet attitude!

Why Is Diet Culture Perilous?

The strain to keep a specific body standard and make rules and guidelines around food can prompt:

- Outrageous limitation in calories
- Feeling regretful in the wake of eating
- Removing nutrition types that can contain fundamental nutrients and minerals (for instance, I eat nothing with sugar).
- Supporting inordinate activity or master ana exercises that can prompt injury, hunger, or low glucose.
- Utilization of purgatives exercise, or cleansing for the discipline of eating food
- Dietary problems
- One of the most widely recognized supporters of cluttered eating is counting calories at an early age.

We should Trench Diet Culture!

The following are 8 hints to jettison diet culture:

- Call out fatphobia
- Decline to weigh at medical care visits that aren't therapeutically important
- Quit utilizing marks like great/awful/solid and unfortunate food
- Try not to advance activity for the goal of reshaping the body
- Perceive your own body checking and decrease it
- Be a promoter of weight inclusivity
- Eliminate scales from your home
- Practice delicate nourishment

All of us play a part in destroying diet culture and fatphobia.

Not certain, assuming that you're eating fewer carbs? Take this food opportunity test to find out!

Everybody plays a part in supporting dump diet culture. Assuming you're feeling overpowered in the excursion to discard diet culture, look at these body good diary prompts to assist with supporting you in getting everything rolling. It's likewise smart to keep a rundown of body good certifications close by for when you are feeling overpowered.

Chapter 2

Break The Code Of Emotional Eating

Do you rush to the storage room when you feel down or are generally furious? You're in good company. It's normal for individuals to go to nourishment for solace as a method for adapting to huge, troublesome sentiments.

The point when you eat in light of feelings, it's called emotional eating. Everybody does it at times.

Our bodies need food to make due. It's a good idea that gobbling illuminates the prize framework in the cerebrum and encourages you.

While emotional eating happens frequently, and you don't have alternate ways of adapting, it very well may be an issue.

Even though it might feel like a method for adapting in those minutes, eating doesn't resolve the genuine issue. In the unlikely event that you are feeling

worried, restless, exhausted, desolate, miserable, or tired, food won't fix those sentiments.
For certain individuals, this pattern of going to food to adapt makes responsibility and disgrace — more intense sentiments to explore.
Food is the focal point of such countless things that we do. Food is important for our festivals. Making nourishment for somebody going through an unpleasant time is a method for showing you give it a second thought. Imparting food to others is a method for interfacing.
Having a profound association with food is regular.
The objective is to permit you to settle on a cognizant conclusion about when, what, and how you eat. There will be times when it's a good idea for food to be important for managing huge feelings. At different times, there are better ways of adapting.
their feelings?
Nearly anything can set off a craving to eat. Normal outside purposes behind profound eating might include:

- work pressure
- monetary concerns
- medical problems
- relationship battles

- Individuals who follow prohibitive weight control plans or have a past filled with counting calories are more likely to eat inwardly.

Other potential inward causes include:

- absence of contemplative mindfulness (acknowledging how you feel)
- alexithymia (absence of capacity to figure out, process, or portray feelings)
- feeling dysregulation (powerlessness to deal with feelings)
- switched hypothalamic pituitary adrenal (HPA) stress hub (under-dynamic cortisol reaction to stretch)
- Emotional eating is in many cases a programmed conduct. The more that food is utilized to adapt, the more settled the propensity becomes.
- Is personal eating a dietary problem?
- Emotional eating all alone isn't a dietary problem. It tends to be an indication of cluttered eating, which might prompt fostering a dietary issue.

Confused eating can include:

- being extremely unbending with food decisions
- marking food varieties as "great" or "terrible"
- continuous slimming down or food limitation
- frequently eating because of feelings as opposed to actual appetite
- unpredictable dinner timing
- fanatical considerations about food that begin to impede the remainder of your life
- sensations of culpability or disgrace after eating food varieties you view as "unfortunate"

As indicated by the Institute of Nourishment and Dietetics, dietary problems are analyzed when an individual's eating ways of behaving meet specific measures. Many individuals have confused eating ways of behaving but don't meet the rules for a dietary problem.

You needn't bother with being determined to have a dietary problem to look for help. You have the right to have a decent connection with food.

On the off chance that you figure you might have confused eating ways of behaving, talk with emotional well-being proficient or enlisted dietitian.

Why Food?

There are many justifications for why eating turns into a method for adapting. Troublesome feelings might prompt a sensation of vacancy or a profound void.

Eating discharges dopamine. Dopamine is a mental substance that encourages us.

We additionally foster propensities and schedules with food. Assuming that you generally eat when pushed, you could go after food at the earliest hint of pressure without acknowledging it.

What's more, food is legitimate, and you can get it all over the place. Messages and pictures about food can build your sensation of appetite.

Emotional hunger vs Physical hunger

People should eat to live. It's normal to require food and to want specific preferences or surfaces.

You might consider how to differentiate between emotional and actual craving prompts. It may very well be precarious. Once in a while, it's a mix of both.

On the off chance that you haven't eaten for a few hours, or for the most part don't eat sufficiently in a day, you are bound to encounter profound eating.

Here are a few signs to assist you with differentiating.

Physical hunger	Emotional hunger
Grows gradually over time.	Come on abruptly.
Feel the sensation of fullness and accept it as a prompt to stop eating.	Do not sense the feeling of fullness so it doesn't stop you from needing to eat more.
Attached to the last time you ate.	Triggered by the requirement for solace or calming.

The most effective method to be aware assuming that you're a personal eater

Individuals who experience emotional eating might feel:

- crazy around specific food sources
- a desire to eat when they feel strong feelings
- an inclination to eat in any event, when they are not truly eager
- like food quiets or rewards them.

Chapter 3

Making Peace With Food ….. and Thyself

At the point when you, at last, wipe the slate clean with food, you will presently not be spooky by that cupcake, frozen yogurt, or pasta. Figure out how Standard 3 of Natural Eating: Bury the hatchet with Food, can assist you with putting food distraction behind you.

How frequently do you ponder food?

Assuming you're similar to most people, contemplations of food involve more than the 2-3 hours that specialists consider sound. You could wind up tormented by the treats dish at work or the pastry that you consider undesirable. Or on the other hand, you may be encountering culpability and disgrace about the chips you ate since you buckled after not eating them for a month.

There is another way!

Wiping the slate clean with Food will assist desires, distraction, and binges with becoming a relic of past times.

Frequently, individuals genuinely accept that they allow themselves to eat food varieties. They in all actuality do eat food varieties they view as undesirable or illegal. Be that as it may, it's generally on a "cheat day" or when they disregard one of their food rules. It may very well be eating pastry just at a unique event or at a birthday celebration, or eating a pack of chips in the wake of a difficult day at work.

In any case, how about we survey what burying the hatchet with food is:

- Reconciling with food implies giving yourself Unqualified consent to eat ALL food varieties.
- The word genuine is vital to reconcile with food.
- Genuine is characterized as "not exposed to any circumstances."
- Consider it: Do you give yourself unrestricted consent?
- Or on the other hand, in the same way as other of the ladies with whom I work….
- Do you just permit a specific serving size?
- Do you utilize exercise to make up for eating specific food varieties?
- Do you have sensations of culpability or disgrace?
- Do you possibly permit food varieties when you are at a specific weight
- Do you have rules about when or how frequently you can eat these food sources?

On the off chance that you replied "yes" to any of the inquiries above, you are putting conditions around your eating encounters. Also, eventually, this will keep you from reconciling with food and accomplishing the delight that accompanies turning into an instinctive eater. Frequently, I hear regrets like "I have zero control over myself around Doritos. Assuming that I eat one, I eat the entire pack." When I request that potential clients challenge this reasoning, they give me substantial instances of binging as well as binging on these "terrible" food sources. Anyway, there is consistently a steady in this story:

Hardship.

These prohibited food varieties have been confined or missing from diets, or "clean eating" regimens. After a time of swearing off these food varieties, the desire for this food increases until you begin pondering it constantly. It very well may be seven days, a month, or a year, yet when you eat the food, you begin eating it in enormous amounts. Sensations of responsibility and disgrace emerge as you swear you'll backpedal on your eating regimen (or "good dieting plan") tomorrow.

Amusingly, even as you're eating this food that you've been desiring, you're not appreciating it since you're anticipating your looming diet. Your brain realizes that this food will be missing from your eating routine for a period, so you're "getting your fill" today before the hardship begins once more.

For some ladies, this hardship, hankering, gorge, disgrace cycle continues endlessly for quite a long time. It could appear to be unique: Some call it a cheat day, while others go for broadened periods without the food, however eventually, it's no different either way.

You, as countless ladies, probably won't know that you're doing it since "food rules" and hardship are so applauded by our general public. Furthermore, the disgrace that follows a gorge isn't something that we will quite often examine with others. It very well may be a propensity that you could have been uninformed about. Maybe, that is no joke "aha" second at present…

The excellence of Natural Eating is that you at last restore entrust in your body. All food varieties become impartial: an apple is ethically identical to a piece of chocolate cake since you realize that you can openly have either at whatever point you need.

With Natural Eating, there's no such thing as a cheat day!

Show Me the Evidence!

Maybe this all sounds interesting however you believe some science should back up the hypotheses of hardship and binging.

Our bodies have a base drive to keep our species flourishing. Whenever they are given hardship, our bodies get smart:

Natural variables like expanded hunger chemicals and mental changes make us ponder food. These cycles guarantee that our bodies get the energy we want.

There have been bunches of the way of talking of late about sugar dependence, and so forth. I'll intend to address that in a later blog, yet I will address the science behind hardship.

During The Second Great War, a gathering of faithful dissenters consented to partake in a "starvation study" directed by scientist, Ancel Keys. This gathering of solid men without any set of experiences of eating less junk food were exposed to a period where their calorie admission was sliced to half of their typical admission. Following a half year (and huge weight reduction), their standard eating regimens were continued.

The outcomes were faltering:

Indeed, even after they had restored all the shed pounds, they were fixated on food and detailed dreaming about it, hankering food sources, and in any event, understanding cookbooks (and recall, this was in the 1940s - in a period before The Food Organization)! These impacts continued long after the review had finished.

Constrained hardship (eating less junk food) is the number of ladies that become caught in this hardship - gorge culpability disgrace cycle, yet at times there are different reasons:

Food weakness - When cash is tight, in youth or the present, the powerlessness to buy food varieties can cause sensations of hardship that later result in binge and binging when these food sources are free.

Severe food rules in your group of beginning - A few guardians accept that they are helping their children when they license no treats in the house. Be that as it may, these guidelines frequently blowback when kids are presented with illegal food varieties at school, eateries, or companions' homes. Think about what these children do when they go to the everyday scheduled play date.

These are all kinds of ways that individuals stall out in this cycle.

Anyway, how would you deal with Rule 3 of Instinctive Eating? How would you reconcile with food?

The following are 5 Basic Ways Of burying the hatchet with Food:

- Begin by making a rundown of food sources that you don't eat. I suggest positioning these food varieties from those that incite minimal uneasiness to the most.
- Pick one of these food varieties and buy enough for various servings. No single-serving sacks here.
- Plan an opportunity to eat this food without interruption. Figure out an opportunity when you are very much refreshed and not under loads of pressure.
- Plunk down to eat this food with your faculties as a whole. Note any sentiments that emerge: nervousness, disgrace, responsibility, satisfaction, and so forth. You might view journaling about the experience as supportive.

Proceed with this cycle until this food turns out to be genuinely unbiased.

Many individuals enjoy inquiries concerning making harmony with food and how to start the interaction.

Here are the main 4 inquiries that I get posed in regards to wiping the slate clean with food:

1. **Is it that basic?** All things considered, yes. In any case, I genuinely comprehend the feelings of dread and difficulties that show up with this cycle. Mentally, the cycle is basic, yet inwardly, it can require investment and need help. That is the reason many clients work with me, as they get the help of an Enlisted Dietitian as they are going through this interaction. The help is vital to their progress in remaining on the way to turning into a natural eater and halting the hardship gorge cycle.

2. **What amount of time will it require to deal with every food?** This cycle is profoundly individualized so I could do without putting a number on it. By and large, the longer a food has been taboo, the more it will take for that food to turn out to be genuinely impartial. The vast majority of my clients let me know that it's a more limited time when they are being upheld with somebody like me.

3. How numerous servings would it be a good idea for me to permit? I encourage you not to put any limitations around how much of this food you can eat because that will at last proceed with your feeling of hardship. However, my suggestion is to buy more than you naturally suspect you want.

4. **Could I at any point avoid this step yet figure out how to be a natural eater?** To put it plainly, no. I truly comprehend how testing it tends to be to make this stride. Once in a while, I compare it to hopping into the center of the sea without a daily coat. However, without reconciling with ALL food sources, it truly is difficult to break the hardship - gorge cycle you are in at the present moment.

Utilizing the means above can act as your manual for start deliberately managing your trepidation of food varieties to wipe the slate clean with food, a critical stage to turning into an Instinctive Eater

Chapter 4

Free yourself from the past and change your present

Acknowledge, then, at that point, act. Anything the current second contains, embrace maybe you had picked it. This will phenomenally change for what seems like forever." ~Eckhart Tolle

Being available. It sounds so straightforward, isn't that so?

Be that as it may, again and again, we are removed from the current second. Our heads get jumbled with the brain jabber of yesterday, broken recollections, and nerves and fears of what's to come; meanwhile, we look past the excellence and effortlessness of the present — this second, at this moment.

It's taken me years to figure out how to buy and live. My life as a youngster was horrible; my mom died when I was a decade old. I recall the days when I'd visit her at the clinic, gullibly accepting that all was eventually great.

At the point when she passed on, my entire world disintegrated. For quite a long time I lost myself in melancholy, segregating myself to attempt to comprehend what I was feeling. I felt like nobody comprehended me and dreaded the void I felt would consume me until it turned into an ordinary, regular inclination.

I grew up with my dad and six siblings, and it was both a gift and a revelation. Although we're an affectionate family, being the main young lady with no protective impact made it hard for me to embrace my gentility, feel enabled, fabricate certainty, and love myself completely.

I've needed to do a great deal of soul-looking and learning through others and encounters to comprehend who I am and where I'm going.

On account of the extraordinary encounters and feelings from before, it was simple for me to slip once again into old approaches to being, rehash comparative encounters in my day-to-day existence, circumvent around and around — and miss the present.

Figuring out how to acknowledge myself and my past and embrace my present and what's to come as opposed to dreading it has been a nonstop yet productive excursion for me so far.

So here are a few hints I've accumulated along my way, to ideally help and move you to live more comprehensively and presently. blem now or in any case work on the ongoing second. Investing energy zeroed in on what might occur down the line denies you completely encountering what's going on at this point. Life at the time moves rapidly — don't miss it.

1. Recognize the truth about the past.

Figuring out how to acknowledge your past is an interaction, and is generally difficult, especially on the off chance that it was horrible or tragic. To begin with, you want to permit yourself to perceive the truth about your past. Recognize your considerations and sentiments, without judgment; there is no off-base or right method for doing this.

As you disentangle everything to see and gain from quite a while ago, you might need to twist up in a ball and store it all away once more; this is typical. Recollect that tolerating your past isn't tied in with needing to change or just drop it; it's tied in with modifying your view of it so you can live more openly.

When I did this, I needed to acknowledge that my mom wasn't returning. Albeit that was challenging for me, this underlying step liberated me.

From that point forward, I've understood I feel her around enthusiastically, although I can't see her truly, and this is overwhelmingly significant for me. Notwithstanding, I could encounter that after I acknowledged her passing for what it was, and that required a decent two or three years.

The second you start to acknowledge the past is the second you start your mending process. This is the beginning of giving up, continuing, and living something else for the present. Give yourself time. Recollect that this is an interaction, not a race or a rivalry.

2. Check out your feelings.

I can't communicate enough that it is so critical to permit yourself to feel transparently and openly, consistently. Holding onto your feelings, especially the pessimistic ones, just brings more personal unrest and keeps you caught before.

At the point when my mom died, I frequently felt desolate and would clutch that forlornness as an approach to feeling nearer to her. In any case, I find looking back that this pulled me away from others and kept me trapped in a pattern of misery and unreasonable assumptions.

Share how you're feeling with somebody near you, whether it's a companion, relative, accomplice, or specialist; and if you don't have anybody sufficiently close to doing this with, let your feelings out through a non-verbal means.

This could mean getting your guitar and playing a portion of your main tunes, laying out an image, or composing a sonnet. Being inventive is an extraordinary and therapeutic approach to delivering anything that is stuck inside.

I did a blend of these things all through my life as a youngster, and everyone assisted me with becoming mindful of my sentiments, figuring them out, and letting them go.

3. Practice care.

Being careful means monitoring your inward world (your contemplations, feelings, substantial sensations, breathing), and your external world (your environmental factors/climate, activities toward others) with the goal that you can live more as of now.

You can begin a basic care practice by zeroing in exclusively on your breathing; relax for four seconds in, and four seconds out, and do this for around five minutes (you can do this for longer on the off chance that you have additional time).

This is a fast and fabulous method for quieting or stopping the gap in your mind and loosening up your body. What's more, in particular, it's an extraordinary method for taking you back to the current second.

Noticing your contemplations (and how they're affecting you) is another extraordinary care workout. Our brain can invoke countless various contemplations in practically no time. A portion of these contemplations can be positive, others can be negative; however more often than not our considerations are past or future-situated.

Our contemplations make our world. The more you think about a specific idea, the more it turns into an instilled conviction, so it's vital to know about your viewpoints so you manifest a positive reality, not one that is loaded with battle.

As far as I might be concerned, personal torment appeared in medical problems, and I upgraded my battle by letting myself know I was unable to improve. Through care, I figured out how to calm these negative contemplations. While clinical therapy worked on my well-being, I realized my psychological state assumed a critical part in both my disorder and recuperation.

Being in nature can likewise pull you back to the current second. Remove 30 minutes from your day to take a walk or sit outside to be among the trees or your nursery

Notice the sounds you hear — the stirring of the breeze in the trees, the crunching sound of leaf litter, birds trilling, and bugs humming together as one. Taking note of these things and the sentiments or contemplations that accompany these sounds can assist you with recollecting the excellence and effortlessness of the present.

At the point when I take strolls, I help myself to remember these things: the ground is my spirit, the trees are my regular excellence, and the sun is my internal brilliance. Nature is an ideal impression of what your identity is. Submerging yourself in it tends to be a certainty promoter, as well as a wonderful sign of how astounding you are.

Chapter 5

Winning The Tug Of War(How to stop emotional eating)

It tends to be difficult to improve on a propensity like emotional eating, yet it is conceivable. The following are far to assist you with adapting;.

Create An Emotional Journal

The more you figure out your propensities, the better. Eating in light of feeling can happen consequently. The more you comprehend how you feel when you do specific things, the better your opportunity to change things.

Have a go at tracking those times when you eat but are not genuinely eager. Make a note of:

- what was going on
- how you were feeling
- any feelings you saw when you got the desire to eat
- You may likewise need to incorporate a spot to compose what you did. Did you consume right? Did you stand by for a couple of moments? Did you effectively occupy yourself?

Do whatever it takes not to pass judgment on yourself on your discoveries. Attempt to be inquisitive about what's going on when you eat in light of feelings.

This takes a ton of training. Be caring to yourself as you begin to investigate. It doesn't need to be great.

Change Unhealthy Habits

On the off chance that you're accustomed to eating because of profound circumstances, what could you at any point do all things being equal? For a beginning, make a rundown of exercises you could partake in that don't include getting ready, eating, or looking for food. One of the most straightforward, least demanding, and best options in contrast to profound eating is strolling: ordinary strolling, speed strolling, strolling on a treadmill, or strolling your canine. Make exercises like sewing or felting not just take a break and give you something physical to do, yet permit you to be innovative and useful.

When you have more data about the feelings, circumstances, or considerations that can set off eating, you can begin to make changes.

Assuming you notice that you generally eat when you feel anxious, the pressure needs consideration. Ponder a few things you can improve to ease your pressure.

Assuming that you notice you eat when you're exhausted, consider ways of dealing with your weariness. How else might you occupy your time?

It requires investment and practice to move your attitude from going after food to taking part in different exercises. Try different things with various things to find what works for you.

Get to the point of eating and noticing your hunger
We realize that being close to home and having actual cravings can be altogether different things. Be that as it may, ensuring you are getting to the point of eating is a significant foundation propensity.
Our cerebrums are wired to ensure we eat enough for endurance. You might see that you get more desires later in the day on the off chance that you haven't eaten sufficiently that day.
Many individuals observe that eating different food varieties with their feasts is the most fulfilling. You can analyze to see what dinners are most filling for you.
Assuming you observe that you are very hungry during the day, adding more protein might help. Protein sources might keep you feeling more full for longer. Go for the gold out of your day-to-day admission.
Protein sources include:

- meat, poultry, fish, fish
- eggs
- dairy items
- soy refreshment, tofu, tempeh
- beans and lentils
- nuts and seeds

Assuming that you've been now and again abstaining from food for a lot of your life, it tends to be difficult to tune into your yearning and completion signs. It can take training to begin to see what actual cravings and completion feel like.

Monitoring actual craving signals can assist you with seeing when you are eating for emotional reasons.

A few indications of actual craving include:

- stomach rumbling
- feeling discombobulated or insecure
- a drop in energy level
- trouble focusing
- changes in temperament
- expansion in considerations about food

If you might want to reconnect with your craving and completion, picture your yearning for a size of one to ten.

Level one is outrageous yearning. You might feel really unwell, powerless, and prepared to get whatever could be palatable. Ten is outrageous totality, as after a monster occasion feast.

Try to check in with yourself like clockwork and ask yourself what your craving level is. This can assist you with seeing your regular themes of appetite and completion.

As you get more practice, you might begin to see a portion of the early indications of craving. It can likewise assist you with distinguishing when you want to eat yet are not truly ravenous.

Seek for Help

Organization of loved ones, remembering proficient assistance for the type of specialist or mentor, if vital, can be as essential to your prosperity as your inspiration and endeavors. The individuals who care about your prosperity can help by applauding you, sharing thoughts for better feasts, perceiving the emotional eating underpinnings of your binging issues, and maybe in any event, assisting with diffusing a portion of the profound circumstances that trigger your indulging. Encircle yourself with individuals ready to listen closely, offer support and inspiration, or perhaps participate as cooking, strolling, or exercise mates.

Oppose segregation in snapshots of misery or uneasiness. Those are intense sentiments to explore all alone. Indeed, even a speedy call to a companion or relative can do wonders for your state of mind. There are likewise formal care groups that can help.

One self-detailed pilot study by a trusted Source discovered that social help and responsibility assisted the members with better sticking to eating-related conduct change.

Think about getting additional assistance from experts.

Search for a dietitian with experience supporting individuals with emotional or cluttered eating. They can assist you with distinguishing eating triggers and tracking down ways of overseeing them.

A psychological well-being proficiency can assist you with tracking down alternate ways of adapting to troublesome feelings as you create some distance from utilizing food. They frequently utilize mental social treatment (CBT). Ensure you have loved ones who can keep you sure and centered amid stress. It can truly assist you with adhering to a sound way of life. Research shows that individuals with high-stress occupations have better emotional well-being at the point at which they have solid encouraging groups of people.

Organize Your Meals

Eating routinely planned feasts and, for certain individuals, consistently booked snacks, can forestall indulging on the off chance that you adhere to the timetable. Then again, sporadic dietary patterns ordinarily mean something bad since they bring about irregular eating and binging. The vast majority, taking everything into account, plan three dinners and a couple of bites or "smaller than usual feasts" at explicit times. Genuine craving ordinarily kicks in beginning around three hours after your last dinner. Contingent upon your dietary patterns and the hour of the day, a little tidbit might be adequate by then; on the off chance that not, you're getting a sign that it's the ideal opportunity for your next feast.

CBT for emotional eating frequently incorporates conduct techniques, like eating standard dinners at an arranged time. Planning your feasts can assist with checking actual cravings. The feeling of feeling full may likewise assist with

controlling emotional eating cravings.

Some call this the cool hot compassion hole. In the virus state (meaning you're not eager and hence nonpartisan or "cold" toward food), you underrate how hungry you may be from here on out. While in the hot state, you misjudge how hungry you are (emotional eating).

Arranging your feasts might assist with keeping you in a colder or more unbiased state.

In one study, dinner arranging was connected with food assortment, diet quality, and less heftiness.

Planning your dinners doesn't mean you want to prepare seven days of food. All things being equal, consider building a week-by-week feast plan that incorporates breakfast, lunch, supper, and a bite. Then, at that point, conclude what time you will eat every dinner. For example:

Meal	Day of the week	Time
Breakfast	Monday-Friday	7am
Snack	Monday-Friday	10:30pm
Lunch	Monday-Friday	2pm
Dinner	Monday-Friday	6pm
Breakfast	Saturday-Sunday	9am
Lunch	Saturday-Sunday	12pm
Snack	Saturday-Sunday	3pm
Dinner	Saturday-Sunday	6:30pm

Assuming you experience a profound longing to eat, ponder your next booked feast. It might just be a half hour away. Inquire as to whether you can hold back to eat.

Do whatever it takes not to plan dinners excessively near sleep time, and keep every one of your feasts inside a 12-hour window, from 7:00 a.m. to 7:00 p.m. This implies you ought to eat a feast about like clockwork.

Eliminate Distraction

You are eating while you're working or sitting in front of the television, your cerebrum passes up the full eating experience. If conceivable, offer food your full consideration when you eat. This can expand the happiness you get from the food.

At the point when you feel fulfilled, you might be less inclined to search for something different a short time later. Eliminate the desire to nibble on unfortunate food varieties by keeping them out of your home. Stressed over settling on terrible decisions when you shop? Adhere to a severe staple

rundown of good food sources, and never visit the supermarket when you're eager or feeling terrible.
At the point when you are diverted, you are additionally bound to eat quicker. It requires investment for your stomach to tell your cerebrum you're full. On the off chance that you're a quick eater, you might be eating an overabundance before your cerebrum can advise you to stop.
This could be due to molding like Pavlov's canine. One social procedure psychological well-being experts use to adapt to this molding is upgrade control. Improvement control works by changing your food signals.
Most profound eaters feel frail over their food desires. At the point when the inclination to eat hits, it's the sum of everything on your mind. You feel a practically excruciating strain that requests to be taken care of, at present! Since you've attempted to oppose before and fizzled, you accept that your self-discipline simply isn't satisfactory. Yet, in all actuality, you have more control over your desires than you suspect.
Take 5 preceding you yield to a hankering
Profound eating will in general be programmed and essentially careless. Before you even acknowledge what you're doing, you've gone after a tub of frozen

yogurt and finished a portion of it. Yet, if you can pause for a minute to stop and reflect when you're hit with hankering, you offer yourself the chance to settle on an alternate choice.

Develop a positive inner voice

To find success, you want to trust in yourself and remain propelled by a continuous conviction that you can achieve anything you set off to do. You can't be blissful and effective constantly; that is not practical. However, you can figure out how to zero in on your victories, not on your disappointments. You can drive yourself to continue looking for arrangements instead of losing trust or surrendering when you hit a snag. Others can serve generally, however, it depends on you to find your assets and use them to accomplish the inward work, the emotional work that no one but you can do.

self-talk, and self-empathy are more apparatuses to use on your excursion to deal with c
emotional eating. Further developing restorative eating has been shown.
Attempt to turn out to be more mindful of the narratives you are telling yourself. It very well might be useful to record a portion of the rehashed negative considerations you are having.
Recollect that you don't want to trust all that your cerebrum tells you. Become inquisitive about where these contemplations may come from.When you are more mindful of the relative multitude of negative considerations that appear, you can begin to deal with evolving them. Make notes on how you could have an impact on how you converse with yourself. Consider how you would converse with a dear companion and utilize that language with yourself. Try not to fixate on your disappointments. All things considered, gain from your mix-ups. Try not to allow a couple of stumbles to make more pressure. All things considered, center around the 10,000-foot view and perceive how you can break your pressure-eating cycle.
The following are a couple of models:

Rather of	Try
I'm horrible at my job	Everyone has difficulties at work. How might I feel more sure about my job?
Once more,I binged.I'll always be unable to change!	I can't help thinking about why that recurred.
I can't accept that wreck again.	We all commit errors. This is something I can learn from.

Try mindfulness

Mindfulness has many advantages for psychological wellness. It's shownTrusted Source to be a strong method for overseeing nervousness and misery. It has additionally been displayed to diminish pressure eating.

Mindfulness is the act of focusing on the second you are in. Assuming you track down that pressure, low mindset, or uneasiness are triggers for your eating, care practices might help.

Here are a few instances of mindfulness rehearses:

- sitting unobtrusively and zeroing in on your breath
- doing a body sweep to see any areas of strain and deliberately loosening up them
- pay attention to a directed contemplation
- center around the things around you and name a couple of things that you can taste, smell, see, contact, and hear
- Careful eating is an approach to eating that depends on interior prompts to come to conclusions about food. Careful eating is a compelling method for working on your relationship with food and is related to mental prosperity.

It's an approach to encounter the demonstration of eating completely. It urges you to dial back and be more mindful of the food's appearance, smells, flavors, surfaces, and sounds.

Careful eating is tied in with stopping before eating to completely investigate what is required at that point. Is it food? Provided that this is true, what kind of food? On the off chance that not food, what will address this issue?

It requires persistence and investment to figure out how to be a careful eater. To more deeply study, consider working with a dietitian who has insight into careful or natural eating.

Chapter 6

Stop The Damage

The Pattern of Profound Eating When we comprehend emotional eating on a profound level, we can start to recover the power from the cycle. We like to give names to each stage, so they're more straightforward to recognize when they occur in our regular routines. There are four primary phases of...

The Pattern of Emotional Eating Eating

At the point when we comprehend emotional eating on a profound level, we can start to recover the power from the cycle. We like to give names to each stage, so they're more straightforward to recognize when they occur in our day-to-day routines.
There are four fundamental phases of profound eating: trigger, concealment, bogus rapture, and headache.

Trigger: A "trigger" is an occasion or circumstance that causes an upsetting or excruciating emotional reaction. It very well may be any article, occasion, or discussion. Triggers make an actual reaction in the body. Our breathing might accelerate or become shallow, or we might begin perspiring. Inwardly, we could feel irate, miserable, or irritated. Why we have specific triggers rather than others has to do with our family backgrounds, our characters, and generally, our uncertainties.

Conceal: There are numerous ways of concealing sentiments we would rather not feel, yet one of the most widely recognized ways is to eat food sources high in sugar, starches, and fat, for example, frozen yogurt, cakes, and treats. These exemplary solace food varieties are suitably named because they conceal troublesome sentiments by creating a flashing good feeling. Exemplary solace food varieties are weighty and hard to process. Aside from the mind, assimilation requests the most energy. Weighty food varieties pull energy from the sensory system, where we feel our sentiments, and direct it toward processing. These food sources conceal feelings, desensitizing sentiments that began the profound eating cycle in any case.

Bogus Delight: When you gobble to conceal your sentiments, you enter the "misleading rapture" stage. Qualities of this stage are an impression that all is great, that there was no issue to manage in any case, or that it was only a fabrication of your creative mind. The solace food matched with the longing to conceal empowers us to neglect, essentially for a brief time.

Headache: Soon, the impression of ecstasy and neglect begins to wear off and the "headache" sets in. Two sorts of torment happen during the headache. First, there is the actual aggravation and uneasiness, which happens in the wake of eating an over-the-top "solace" food. Then there is the emotional agony, which comes from feeling responsibility and disgrace about not doing what you had initially decided to do (eat clean), rehashing a very much worn design. Additionally, you can frequently feel confused, because you have neglected or stifled the first trigger that began the descending cycle in any case.

Another Trigger: The responsibility and disgrace delivered by the headache frequently go about as another trigger. Then the profound eating cycle starts once more. We keep on eating ineffectively, and the cycle proceeds. As opposed to drawing expanded energy from sound propensities, we feel the converse, a negative cycle that twisting us descending. Large numbers of us imagine that we simply need discipline. In any case, truly we're trapped in the cycle.

Breaking the Cycle Of Emotional Eating

There are no enchanted shots. Breaking liberated from the pattern of profound eating starts with understanding the example and conceding to remembering it when it appears. The cycle might keep on occurring, however, you will turn out to be quicker at seeing and interfering with it when it does.

The following are four methods for breaking the cycle:

Fabricate mindfulness. Mindfulness is the first and most significant stage. With consideration, you will look into the manners in which you and by utilizing this cycle and the narratives and games you play to try not to focus on what you truly care about.

Address the issue straightforwardly. The least difficult and most direct method for interfering with the cycle is to resolve the issue straightforwardly when you feel set off. Frequently profound eating examples can be halted abruptly when the underlying triggers are tended to truly. If you can't talk straightforwardly to an individual, or the trigger is an item, similar to an old image of a family member or the recollections of an accomplice, pause for a minute to completely feel what you are feeling. The mindfulness that you are being set off, in addition to the consent to completely feel what you feel, will decrease the force of the cycle.

Fabricate a tool kit of solid propensities. As well as resolving the issue straightforwardly, subbing a sound propensity for an unfortunate one is the following stage. With cognizant practice, this "tool compartment" will turn out to be more programmed, and we will find your more established propensities falling endlessly normally. You can dive more deeply into these propensities by paying attention to the digital broadcast, however, a couple of our top picks are going for a stroll, drinking a major glass of water, or eating a perfect tidbit.

Get to the root: At the point when certain propensities are not working for us, when they cause us agony and hold us back from advancing toward our objectives, time should be taken to attempt to comprehend and ponder them. Getting to the root implies asking ourselves a few profound inquiries concerning for what reason we do the things we do.
This is a major point that isn't generally effectively settled, however, we feel that tending to here, although it's past the extent of this newsletter, is significant. Investing some energy in considering your propensities, perusing some great self-improvement books, and working with a mentor or specialist can assist you with revealing the more profound motivations behind why you're set off in any case.

6 Lifestyle choices At THE Time

"Living at the time" has propelled many persuasive banners and Shirts, however, it's a significant idea. You've presumably heard a few varieties: Live like crazy. Live as though this will be your last day. Living at the time takes practice, yet when you figure out how to experience along these lines, you will carry on with a more full existence and value the magnificence in each movement all day long. Figure out how to live at the time with these six thoughts.

1. Center Around THE At this point

To live at the time, you want to zero in on the at this point. Center around the thing you're doing. Stop the television, switch off the PC, dial back, and appreciate the present. Alludes to this as care or being with your viewpoints as they are. As per living for the second by rehearsing care decreases pressure, helps your resistant framework, brings down circulatory strain, and has other gainful physical and mental impacts. Dixit adds that careful individuals are safer, have higher confidence, and are more. Enjoying and savoring life at the time — whether it's eating dinner, drinking some espresso or strolling to the store — evokes bliss and other positive feelings.

2. Focus On THE Little THINGS

Notice your general surroundings: the little things. Be grateful for them. Living for the second and considering the little things will assist you with developing more sure encounters. You focus on the easily overlooked details that satisfy you, such as eating frozen yogurt, blowing air pockets, or paying attention to music, as these things can have an enormous effect on the way you feel.

3. Grin

If you have any desire to know how to live at the time, you simply need to investigate the mirror and grin. Grin — it can impact how you feel. There is a relationship in our psyche between how we feel and how we respond. On the off chance that we feel blissful, we grin. Assuming we grin, it encourages us. Our face imparts our perspective to other people and ourselves. So grin — it will make you more joyful and assist you with valuing life at the time.

4. PERFORM Arbitrary Thoughtful gestures

Arbitrary thoughtful gestures, those benevolent demonstrations that help other people, assist you with living for the snapshot of making others grin and making you grin too. Arbitrary thoughtful gestures are only that — irregular. They are unconstrained, at the time, and an incredible expansion to your day-to-day existence.

The following time you see that individual strolling in the downpour, offer them your umbrella. That abandoned driver? Call for help. The old woman battling with her food? Convey them for her. One of the simplest examples of how to live at the time is to work on something for another person without anticipating anything consequently. It assists you with living at the time but works on that second for yourself and another person.

5. Express appreciation

Be grateful. Sounds simple, right? However, it isn't dependable. It doesn't need to be Thanksgiving for you to feel appreciative and offer that thanks.

Occasionally, make sure to pause and consider exactly the way that you have it. At the point when your companion makes you grin, express gratitude toward her for being a major part of your life. At the point when your supervisor gives you another undertaking, express profound gratitude, recollecting that you have some work and can put food on the table. At the point when you think it or feel it, say it right then. Live at the time by offering your thanks when you feel it.

6. Sit back and relax

It's a lot harder than it sounds, yet attempt to recall that stressing today won't change what happens tomorrow. Consistently you spend in stress over what's in store is a moment of the present squandered. Since stressing removes you from this second and transports you into the domain of prospects, living at the time and stress simultaneously is inconceivable.

All things considered, assuming conditions are alarming, center around ways you can tackle a current issue now or in any case work on the ongoing second. Investing energy zeroed in on what might occur down the line denies you completely encountering what's going on at this point. Life at the time moves rapidly — don't miss it.

Chapter 7

How Living As of now Can Guarantee A Brilliant Future

Since you have a thought of how you can live by and by, it's tied in with rehearsing these things routinely so you can guarantee your future is brimming with light as opposed to dread and old examples.

They say that the current second is all we have, and keeping in mind that our past and future are genuine ideas, they are simply different parts of this at this point. Feeling dread and uneasiness toward our future comes from dismissing our present and clutching our past — so to partake in our future, we should initially figure out how to partake in our present!

You are precisely who you should be and where you should be at this time. Wishing or attempting to be another person or elsewhere just makes protection from the present.

So permit yourself an opportunity to acknowledge your past, feel straightforwardly and uninhibitedly, and practice care — and realize that thusly, you're not just living as of now, you're likewise making the most ideal future for yourself.

8 Moves toward Get away From the Past You Want to Abandon.

I've had a lot of restless evenings. Evenings when I was so stressed over something that had occurred in the past that I let it direct my future. We've all been there eventually. You're in good company.

I'm discussing those times when we can't shake the past. Whether it's something little, such as establishing a horrendous first connection or saying something you wish you hadn't, to something significant, such as having to close your business. Nagging negative encounters is difficult and, when we clutch that aggravation, we can't continue toward something more sure.

That is the reason you must let it proceed to abandon the past with these eight strategies.

1. Gain from an earlier time however doesn't abide there.

Indeed. Those negative encounters you had can be utilized for learning and future encounters - - regardless of how difficult they are. Carve out the opportunity to consider the experience and take a gander at ways it can help you not too far off.

You can gain from your encounters by considering these couple of straightforward inquiries:

What truly occurred? Answer exclusively by defying current realities.

What feelings do I feel? I for one prefer to get them on paper.

How can I use this to better myself and my feelings?

In the wake of responding to these inquiries, now is the ideal time to continue. While considering the past for a tad of time is OK, harping on it will just keep those pessimistic considerations and sentiments around.

2. Put yourself out there.

Make it a point to the aggravation you're feeling off your mind. Whether conversing with the individual who has hurt you (or who you hurt), venting to a companion, or getting it on paper, communicating your sentiments can help you in figuring out what, regardless, should be finished to continue.

All the more significantly, it's great for your well-being. Clutching your sentiments prompts uneasiness, wretchedness, cerebral pain, and hypertension. A saying says "When now is the right time to communicate your sentiments, make a point to utilize "I" messages. Portray the level of your feelings, and offer them to somebody who will tune in and not condemn. This will assist you with communicating the melancholy you're not kidding."

3. Quit pointing fingers.

Assuming the part of the casualty is simple and once in a while feels better, particularly contrasted and tolerating reality. The problem is, that blaming others prevents you from moving forward. Most frequently, it is simply grumbling to point fingers. A saying says, "When we fail, we naturally enter the negative zone. We severely dislike another person or some outer variable since we couldn't form life into our approval."

4. Center around the present.

One of the best ways of relinquishing the past is to embrace the present. Rather than remembering the past and getting consumed with cynicism, keep yourself dynamic and partake in the ongoing second. Become familiar with another ability. Reflect. Work out. Eat with a companion. Make another companion. Anything it is, simply live at the time - regardless of whether it's sitting at your work area and watching the mists roll by. I for one "adapt" by building my business and the fate of eCash. It spurs me and helps give me something to dedicate my life towards.

Living at the time, likewise referred to care as, "includes being with your viewpoints as they are, neither getting a handle on them nor driving them away." Brain science Today asserts that those who exercise caution are happier and more jubilant, more compassionate, and safer."

To accomplish a more careful state, know about the thing you are thinking and feeling, lessen reluctance, search out new encounters and acknowledge your gloomy sentiments and circumstances as just being a piece of life.

5. Separate for some time.

Permit yourself to remove some time with the goal that you can clear your head. You don't need to go hiking through Europe. Simply eliminate yourself from the circumstance by limiting any association with individuals, spots, and things that help you to remember the past. Rehearsing ways of separating for some time will allow you the opportunity to encounter something positive - - regardless of whether that is simply setting up camp at a nearby camping area with practically no admittance to web-based entertainment.

At the point when you return, you'll have a viewpoint on the past.

6. Ponder individuals around you.

Take stock of individuals around you. Who is negative and continuously cutting you down? Who are individuals related to the past that you're attempting to get away from? You might have to

create some distance from these people to find more sure individuals who will engage you.
There are a very sizable amount of ways of meeting new individuals, for example, going to neighborhood meetups and gatherings. Try not to be timid. Get yourself out there and find another gathering of companions and colleagues who can assist you with pushing ahead.

7. Pardon the individuals who violated you - - including yourself.

Assuming you've been wounded by somebody, the last thing that you might believe should do is pardon them. There are various moves toward assisting you with pardoning somebody, such as embracing the past while continuing, pursuing another concurrence with yourself, not nodding off furious, and being caring and liberal.
In the meantime, pardon yourself. Nobody is perfect,and we all make mistakes. Rather than kicking yourself for your previous mishaps, cut yourself a little leeway and spotlight the illustrations that you've learned.
When you're not conveying that indignation and disdain, you'll have the option to continue.

8. Gain new experiences.

At long last, begin making new, positive recollections to supplant those negative recollections from an earlier time. Invest your energy with individuals who satisfy you, the things that give you pleasure, and in the spots that bring you harmony. Gaining new experiences is better than being caught before.

Conclusion

In conclusion, we have been discussing the 7 techniques you can employ to combat emotional eating and be free from binging.

The aim of this book is to share the 7 techniques to combat emotional eating and be free from binging. From the beginning I have been very clear to share with you these secrets,have I succeeded? We talked about diet culture and what it entails,why it's perilous and ways to to get rid of this culture, I also talked about emotional eating,the causes and why food and also the techniques to combat emotional eating.

These 7 techniques discussed are secrets to combating emotional eating and being free from binging.

Thanks for buying this book;I hope you've enjoyed it. Now you can have some fun putting everything you've learned into practice.

www.ingramcontent.com/pod-product-compliance
Lightning Source LLC
LaVergne TN
LVHW050331160826
845677LV00014B/3587

* 9 7 9 8 3 7 4 3 4 1 1 4 0 *